C000067636

WRITING BACK TO HAPPINESS

How to write the little stories in life

Kay Underdown

A special collaboration with

Jennifer Achner   Heather Carter

Susan Northrop   Jeanie Roberts

WRITING BACK TO HAPPINESS

Kay Underdown

ISBN 978-1-912899-05-0

Published Spring 2022

Cover design Jessica Wakerley

Copyright © Kay Underdown

Copyright in personal contributions included remains with the person contributing. Consent has been given by the contributors for these to be included in this publication and in different formats of the same content and publication title.

All rights reserved. No part of this publication may be reproduced or transmitted in any form or by any means, electronic or mechanical, including photocopying, recording, or any information storage or retrieval system, without the prior express written permission of the author and contributors where appropriate.

The moral rights of the author and contributors have been asserted.

remembering with love

those who live on in our hearts forever

~

sharing together is where magic begins,

time spent in love and friendship is timeless

~

write your life, write your love,

write your dream

Introduction

In January 2019 I ran an eight-week "Life Story Writing" course as part of a local initiative to enrich the lives of the over 50's. It was a rewarding and fascinating experience and in many ways I learned just as much as I taught.

This book tells the story of that group and how sharing and exploring our experiences led us to find positive ways forward and improved our well-being.

In this book I have been able to share some of our many personal accounts, and I have also included some practical suggestions which could get you started, either individually or in a group.

We hope this will inspire you to write your own stories and motivate you to improve your own sense of well-being.

Writing activities

To inspire your Life Story Writing a list of prompts are provided at the end of each chapter. Here are some suggestions for their use but enjoy taking them wherever they lead you *(subject to the important well-being note opposite)*:

1. Choose one prompt from the list, set a timer for five minutes, *just write* and see what ends up on the page *(see Chapter 3)*.

2. Reflect on all the words in the list then *just write* for about twenty minutes *(again see Chapter 3)*.

3. Select three words, imagine you have been given them as an activity to write a little story about your life that you would like to share with others. Spend a week writing and/or drawing your story.

It is recommended that you start off with 1 and 2 above to get used to *just writing*, without correcting or judging your own work, and discover the surprises and magic that can happen when you allow yourself to do this. I use the term *just write* throughout the book for writing without judgement. So, for most of the time, no stopping to correct your spelling, change your mind or cross things out, *just write*.

Important well-being note

If you find that your writing, or any other activity arising from this book, is lowering your mood or upsetting you, please choose a different theme or activity, one that will bring happy thoughts. Think of places that you love or distract yourself immediately by doing something totally different that you know you will really enjoy and return to writing on a different theme later (it's good to think ahead about the different things you could choose to do in such circumstances).

Throughout this book the term *homework* is used, a term that came from the group themselves when they eagerly asked for writing activities that they could do at home. For me, homework reminds me of the many hours I spent sitting at the family dining table before dinner studying for my O levels, I have always enjoyed learning. For others it may have negative connotations, so please choose your own word for the book's activities that you choose to do.

Life exploration activities

Underlying my approach to writing about life is my belief in the value of using a life coaching approach, combined with creativity and exploration of sense of belonging.

I have therefore included a few stand-alone exercises spaced through the book, similar to those I may occasionally bring to my Life Story Writing workshops. They can be done at any time so if you flick through the book and you feel drawn to one, enjoy the journey it takes you on. You can do the same activity more than once as each time it may be a different experience and bring up different results. There's no right or wrong way, it's enjoying the process and the stories that come out of the activities that matter. (For ease of finding, these have a bold **Life exploration activities** heading.)

Life exploration activity no 1

Nature in my life (one hour +)

1. Draw a line across the middle of a sheet of plain paper (landscape position will be best).

2. Mark the far left as **Birth** and the far right as **Now**.

3. Divide the line into three sections and put the headings above each section:

   Child, **Teenager**, **Adult**.

4. Think about when you were a child, what place did nature play in your life, make notes along, on top or under the line, however you wish to do it. Repeat with Teenager and Adult.

5. Use the notes as triggers to write about your journey with nature throughout your life. What memories does this bring up? What stories, people and places? Either set yourself a time limit, (recommended 30 minutes minimum) or take as long as you wish, relaxing into the process.

With grateful thanks to my very special friends

on the Isle of Thanet

a place that I will think of fondly forever

Chapter 1

December 2019

How a day can turn around in a matter of hours. Life is precious, too good to be wasted. Spend time doing the things that really matter, make time for special occasions. They can be planned or unplanned, it matters not, but they are waiting for you to grab hold of.

Each of us is on a different path but we merge in and out with different people. There are times when the universe creates opportunities for a group of people's lives to meet on the same path. Yet that same path is different for each and every one of us … Magic happens when the moments of convergence result in shared experiences of such simplicity yet memorable for life resulting in shared experiences that enrich life itself and the future to come.

Friendship December 2019

Today I'm writing my Christmas cards and the first ones to be written are laid out before me. Four women that came into my life in January 2019, almost a year ago … we have shared such a wealth of personal stories with laughter and tears on such a regular basis and in such a social way. It really feels unique and strong bonds have been created … I feel that the combination of being an all-women group, together with the therapeutic benefits of writing and sharing stories, has made this "thing" that we have between us amazingly special and something to be treasured. Treasured for what it is now and what it may become in the future, a treasured memory.

After a wonderful Christmas celebration that included a fabulous meal, gift giving and sharing stories, it was a throwback comment during a particular moment of jollity that suggested the title of this book. Little did we realise as Christmas approached, that the New Year was going to bring such an unfathomable time. With the looming of the coronavirus pandemic our weekly meetings came to an abrupt halt as we agreed to cancel our next meeting. The following week, in March 2020, the UK went into lockdown.

Whilst this may seem a negative way to start writing a book on happiness, my life coaching approach to Life Story Writing helps people experiencing difficult times, for whatever reason, to find ways to bring increased positivity into their lives. The purpose of this book is to share our writing group's story, along with my Waves and Pebbles approach, so that you may find something that inspires you to either start, or continue, your Life Story Writing journey – either on your own or with a group of friends – and that you may find the coaching approach to sharing stories about life both inspiring and life changing in some way.

Where have we come from and where are we going? March 2020

Little did I know that what had gone before was going to change so radically in such a short time. Since last night we are now in effect in lockdown as a result of the coronavirus so what I write today is different to what I would have written a week ago ... and even more different to two weeks ago when I came up with this title. So, if I had written this two weeks ago then I need to immerse myself in my time travelling box and imagine how I would be feeling now ... this is me, answering the question two weeks ago.

I have come from a family that grew up in Brighton, from a grammar school and then college secretarial education to live in Kent. I ended up spending most of my adult life in Medway, where we had access to the riverside and estuary, and when both my father and mother had passed away, moved to Broadstairs in 2017 with my daughter.

Having followed a secretarial career up until I had my children, including a period commuting to London, I followed a colourful mosaic of a career mainly in the education and social services field. Yet there was nothing creative about my career until my creative thought processes came to bear while managing a mediation service, enabling the opportunity to learn and explore the benefits of creativity when helping people to overcome difficulties in their lives.

Redundancy led to a creative writing course that was to have immense impact on my life in many ways. It was the catalyst for my going to university to study social sciences, leading to my interest in sense of belonging. It reinforced the benefits of creativity and bringing people together to share their stories and experiences. And it gave me a different path ... the one I had been looking for, and this is how I ended up running a Life Story Writing group in Broadstairs.

And where am I going? I am on a creative journey to bring the benefits of writing to a wider audience facilitated by the increased experience and opportunities I have gained through my special writing group. Both the opportunities to write more about random things and seeing the impact on others on their own journey in life. I am headed for a special place that I have yet to find but the very best part of that is the journey.

Where do we come from and where are we going? Sue March 2020

We all know we begin life as babies. My mum told me quite early on that I was found under a gooseberry bush but later when my sister was born we were told Nurse Early brought her. Nurse Early was the midwife who called to the house a few times.

With a bit of practice and a lot of experimenting I soon found out none of the above was true.

Where are we going?

Now that's a difficult question and the answer depends on one's beliefs.

We all know we are going to die but how, when and where? Who knows?

Why – why do some die young while others live to be 100 and more.

As children we believed if we were good we'd go to heaven and if we were bad we'd be sent to the other place.

Where is Heaven – we all have different views. To me, sunshine, a beach and my friends and family around me.

And Hell – where it's cold, no sunshine or living in a block of flats with no outlook.

I hope Barry's in heaven. He should be.

When he was a teenager he lived next door to my friend who tells me he was a goody goody who stayed at home making model airplanes when everybody else were sampling the dance halls and hotspots of Margate … I hope when I go it's not too soon but please promise you'll make sure I have a flattering photo on my Order of Service

and please don't play "I did it my way!"

Where have we come from and where are we going? Heather March 2020

At last I have finally got round to doing my homework for last week, the first of our classes which we have had to postpone because of the virus. I have taken these questions to relate to our group.

When I saw the details of the "Life History Course" … I thought it might be interesting, particularly the writing element, as I thought it might get me involved in a bit of writing. Whilst I had a degree in English Literature, taught English and in later life wrote endless reports, letters, minutes, etc I had not, since the age of about 16 actually written anything creatively and I thought this might be a gentle introduction. To be honest I had no plans to write my life history as, having no children, I doubt whether anyone would be remotely interested once I am gone. I did, however, have a vague idea that having been through the trauma of my husband's progressions through and death from Alzheimer's, somehow writing might help me make sense of my difficult experiences.

I arrived at the Library for the first session and was surprised to find it a very comfortable and relaxed experience. By the end of the second session, we had settled into the group of 5 which has continued on. From the start we actually wrote spontaneously and did homework. In those first two sessions, I found it amazing that I could just write and not feel embarrassed about reading it out loud.

Well where did we all come from? Simplistically we all came from close by ... All of us, remarkably, came from sorrow, loss and trauma. Somehow, we formed a bond very quickly. We didn't dwell endlessly on the tragedies that had befallen us, but we found ourselves in a safe environment where we could talk about what had happened to our loved ones and to ourselves ...

Being able to talk about what had happened and then, ever so gently, being guided outward like the increasing ripples in a pond, meant that we all began to talk about other important parts of our lives and to be ourselves more. We had objects we treasured, we showed off our talents, we laughed at our hoarding, remembered our holidays, and slowly moved forward as ourselves. With Kay's patient, gentle guidance and fascinating interventions we used life wheels to assess our priorities, plan our futures, and value ourselves.

This leads me to where are we going? We are going to get through this horrendous time, because we have managed our own horrendous times and started to put an eye to the future. We've found things that lighten our moods, we've been and still can be, inspired by things as simple as a small flower in a box, a jug, pickle fork and lovely old photos and art works. We will keep in touch online and keep writing and sharing, and when life finally returns to normal, we will, I am sure, start to meet up again and enjoy our Wednesday sessions. My biggest concern is how we will cope without those delicious homemade biscuits – perhaps they could deliver?

My personal experience of this pandemic, especially during the first few weeks when everyone, apart from key workers, were urged to stay at home and schools were closed, somehow took me back to when I was admitted to hospital back in 2015 and diagnosed with Acute Promyelocytic Leukaemia. First, I was confined to the hospital grounds, then to the ward, then to my room and finally to my bed, spending three weeks in the high dependency unit due to a complication caused by the treatment that affected my lungs. Thankfully I came out the other side after a year of treatment and spending quite a number of weeks in hospital. This experience both challenged me yet in a way ended up enriching my life. It left me with a fresh outlook that I might otherwise not have had, and to starting up my Waves and Pebbles blog which then led to my first book "Life Happens Live Happy".

I wrote the following while sitting outside the consultant's room for my six-monthly check-up.

The Frame **May 2019** *As I wandered through the hospital grounds in the warmth of the sun, my homework popped into my head. The Frame. Somehow it had come into my mind to write about the Frame of Life.*

We create different frames for our life and sometimes life itself creates ours. Sometimes they're not quite what we expect and would not be of our choosing, but we're stuck with them. We then have a choice. Reject the frame but it keeps rebounding to knock us back or embrace the frame for what it is and find the right picture to put in it. The right vision of our life in its new frame. One that we can live with and find ways to bring the colours that we love into it. Sometimes we can find a new dream to capture in that unwelcome frame, once we have had time to reflect and discover that it's not so bad after all.

Other times we may feel so lucky. We have the perfect frame with the perfect picture and are just waiting in anticipation for something to smash it as we don't deserve such joy. Yet joy is there for us to capture in our own personal frame. Whether it be the one we choose or that which has landed upon us, shattering our once-held dreams.

Joy can be found in the most unexpected places ... and sometimes ... just sometimes ... it is found outside the frame.

Life exploration activity no 2

Seven little things that bring me joy (30 minutes)

1. List seven little things that bring you joy.

   To help, think about your senses, things you like to see, hear, touch, smell and taste.

   For me, what springs to mind is catching sight of a robin in my garden or enjoying the sensation of a smooth dark chocolate cherry in kirsch at Christmastime.

2. Pick one that you can either experience this week or find a picture or photo and sit down and spend a few mindful moments reflecting on it.

3. Spend five minutes or more writing about it.

10

CHRISTMAS

THE THINGS I LOVE IN MY LIFE

STARS

PETS

A MEMORABLE DAY

TURQUOISE

MY FAVOURITE DESSERT

THE WEEK-END

AN UNEXPECTED PRESENT

A SPECIAL PHOTO

Chapter 2

On a Wednesday morning in January 2019, I turned up to run my first eight-week course on Life Story Writing - Write the Old, Inspire the New. I had designed the course and was delivering it for a local charity aimed at people aged 50+. I myself had been on one of their courses and it helped me gain a sense of belonging in the new area to which I had recently moved. My own course was being held at a local library. Looking back at writing I did on the day, before everyone arrived, I said that I felt destined to be there. How true that has turned out to be.

Enough people had enrolled for it to happen but only four turned up on the rainy day. Three women and one man. The man didn't turn up the following week, but another woman did, making it four women – Heather, Jenny, Jeanie and Sue - the wonderful ladies in my special writing group. At the beginning of the course Heather wrote *"I had no idea what this would entail, but I am really pleased that it has such a positive slant and may help me keep a positive grip on the many, many memories I have of my life, but particularly of Alan."* Towards the end of the course, I asked if the ladies would write something about their experience of being on the course, the following is what they wrote in March 2019.

The time spent with Kay and the ladies have been most enjoyable.

I have discovered things that I had forgotten about. The pleasure found reminiscing has also been enjoyable.

I still want to write my life story for my grandchildren, however long it takes. Maybe a remote island with no interruptions would be ideal. Also one thing leads to another the memory is good at going backwards.

Things have been talked about on the course that make me think of so many "yesterdays". Just the time to remember for longer and put them all down on paper. If I write like I talk no one would see me again!! (Jeanie)

I didn't think I could just sit down and write about anything at all without planning. I have found that a really interesting experience. It is also re-assuring to find that as the pen hits the paper it suddenly opens up little memories and bigger and bigger and sharper memories. Somehow this enables you to recapture happy moments and to better understand the downs too.

I had, I think, previously been hampered by the traditional structures - wondering how you thought of an idea, planned it, structured it and wrote it correctly. This course has enabled me to take a fresh approach and has given me ideas to spark off writing. I'm not yet sure where I want to take the writing, but I definitely want to continue with it. I think the prompts of decades, life wheel, photos and objects are a good starting point. I might try to use my own life experiences - even some of the bits of writing done here - to write a short story - or even a small book of random memories - it would be nice to see them in print if only for myself. (Heather)

"For a long time now I've been thinking I'd like to write about my life and I heard about this course at a point when I was ready to do so.

If I'd been left to my own devices I would probably have started "I was born in Hastings in 1945 ..." By the time anybody reading it reached 1950 they would almost certainly have fallen asleep or put it down.

The course has shown me that there are other ways of writing not necessarily in chronological order but paragraphs or chapters relating to events and experiences that had taken place during my lifetime. So far I've written about nature (my childhood), my dad who was in the airforce.

Miss Jelly - my teacher.

A journey - one taken regularly in Turkey

and more obscure subjects like my shed! (Sue)

When I first decided I would like to do this course I wasn't certain exactly what we would be doing. I think 'life story' attracted me but I suppose I thought it would be a chronological piece for my children to read later on.

However it has been so much more than that. The writing we have done has unlocked many memories and these in turn have indeed been part of my life story. Taking the various suggested topics like work, activities I like doing, going on a journey have all linked to parts of me and my life which are so much more than a list of dates and places. I hope that I can use these topics and others to continue this writing. (Jenny)

Life exploration activity no 3

My life values in pictures (two hours +)

What do you really value in your life? Choose between three and six life values. Examples are health, wealth, family, friends, contribution, humour, creativity, freedom, independence, nature, humour, but there are many more.

Have a go at taking a selection of photos (or finding some existing pictures) to reflect your chosen values. The images may reflect just one value or several. Try to have at least one main image for each value.

1. Use the photos to help you prioritise your values by arranging them in order from most important to least important. (You may discover that it is not as easy as it sounds.)

2. Create a collage with the photos that will provide you with a visual reminder of what is important to you.

3. Reflect on your experience of doing this activity and *just write* for ten minutes.

16

JANUARY

NATURE IN MY LIFE

A WINTER'S MEAL

MY FRIENDS AND ME

A SNOWMAN'S WISH

MY HOPES AND DREAMS

THE MILLENIUM

THE WOODS

DELIGHTS OF THE WINTER EVENINGS

WANDERING

Chapter 3

Learning how to write for short periods of time, without correcting or questioning what you are writing, is the first step in being able to access the therapeutic benefits of putting pen to paper without judging ourselves. During sessions I often use objects as prompts which are pulled out of my bag at the last moment, or the prompt could just be a title or there may be no prompt, to capture thoughts after carrying out the previous activities. Once finished, we take turns to share what we have written. There's no pressure, even the odd few words shared can lead to interesting conversations.

It's important to say that there is no critiquing in any of my groups or courses. The focus is on the personal enjoyment of recalling, writing and sharing of stories, not on the quality or otherwise of the writing. So, there is no right or wrong way, just a mutual respect for everyone involved.

These are some examples of timed writing. Sometimes the shortest of pieces, which may seem to contain little by way of a story, can lead to the longest diverse conversations when shared with the group. They are often a starting point that may lead to a longer piece of writing for homework.

My trio of William Morris design cake tins contain a variety of resources including coloured felt tips, and a tri-coloured sand egg-timer. One day I realised I had forgotten the egg-timer and exclaimed "I don't have an eggcup!" – lending itself to be the next writing prompt.

I don't have an eggcup Jenny

Why is that? When I love eggs? It's because I am so very good at breaking them. I have had many egg cups over the years – very often they have been picked up by Charles from charity shops – never matching of course. Sadly, they have never lived for very long in my hands. I suppose it's because they are very small and get caught up with other crockery in the cupboard and when I pull out a plate an egg cup flies out with it and crashes onto the kitchen tiles. They rarely live to see another day and if they do, they certainly don't survive the next accident. Perhaps I should stick to scrambled or poached eggs in future.

Jug Sue

Jugs would be a good thing to collect. I have a few. I like gravy boats, not really jugs but I like the shape. I love the blue of Kay's jug especially the dark blue at the base. The handle's an interesting shape. I've got a Worthington E jug at home. One of the few things I've kept from The Plough days. I've got a shelf too which was a barrel rest. It has a Fremlin's elephant on the base. It's dark wood but I painted it white but left the base as if anybody in future wanted it, they could take off the paint and restore it to its original finish.

Mud

Well I didn't know when I chose the bit of paper with mud written on it that I was going to go on a journey to a place near Tunbridge Wells. It's not that it was always muddy, but woods often are, especially when the mass of trees shade the ground from being dried out. This was a gem of a place to visit and have fun with small children, in fact with anyone of any age. There was a trail that you could walk along and every so often there were giant swings hanging from the tall trees. How wonderful it was to swing in nature. Even when it was busy there was so much space that it never felt like anyone much was about. There is so much more to mention – I will have to look it up, including a ride back on the river at the beginning or end of the day depending on which way you chose to go. A place we never tired of. Another hidden part of Kent that makes it a special place to explore.

The powers of Google reminded me that this was Groombridge Place where there is now a treetop walk. I wonder if the swings are still there?

Bells in my life November 2019

Well I thought that was a good starting point but to be honest it's not really bringing anything up, perhaps I need a little time to recall. When I think about it as a child our lives were ruled by the bells at school, a sign that lessons were ending, a sign to pack our bags quickly and move quietly and quickly to our next room and learning activity. Sometimes it was a good feeling, the end of a history lesson that at last was finished or if it was a favourite lesson coming up, such as music, cookery or a language. It is a long distant memory. Perhaps the most pleasant memory of bells was when I arrived by cable car at the top of a mountain in Mayrhofen in Austria. It was a beautiful summers day, blue sky, fresh clean air the like of which I had never before experienced and the wonderful sound of the cowbells in the mountainous silence before me. MAGICAL.

Short pieces like this can inspire further stories. Sue could have written a story about The Plough days. Jenny spoke about her relationship with egg cups and talked about her husband's kind gestures. My own piece about bells could have led to a story about my childhood schooldays or it could have been about holidays in Mayrhofen.

I first went to Mayrhofen with my parents, it was wintertime in the snow. I always recall we had a go at skibobbing, sitting low down on little seats with skis. A few months back I managed to get an old film projector working that belonged to my dad. I popped in an old film and you may imagine how I felt on seeing black and white silent footage of me, when I was about 16 years old, with my mum and dad skibobbing. One day I hope to get that transferred to a DVD, a very special find. The next time I went to Mayrhofen was in my twenties with my husband. We booked a really cheap holiday flying from Lydd Airport to Paris and then getting on a coach to Austria. It was a wonderful holiday with many beautiful walks in the sunshine amongst the mountains. Somewhere I may find some writing I did on our walk down the mountain after the beautiful cowbell arrival – quite a different experience!!

When doing timed writing, if you are unable to think of anything to say then *just write "I don't know what to write"* and keep repeating it until something else slips onto the page. The important thing is to keep writing, be kind to yourself and be patient. Sometimes it's the time or the place that is not helping. Find some time when you have peace for yourself and are comfortable, relax and allow yourself to practice. Remember the writing is for you to enjoy revisiting memories, it is not about perfection though this method may well lead to writing you had never imagined you could do.

Sometimes my own timed writing can turn into something quite reflective.

I feel that I am on a journey into the future and I have no idea what the destination is. It's all about life, what has brought me to this point and I am taking it forward.

This year is turning into a time that I was going to say was some kind of crossroads, but now I feel it's more like a sphere. A golden globe of the world opening up to me yet reflecting the treasured memories of a life that is being well-lived. Not with hundreds of materialistic or the usual dreams like having nice car, big house, dream holiday, but with the special moments that open up the variety and depth of the world, a world yet to be discovered. Yet this year is also about capturing the stories of the past, both my own and others. To savour the delights of past living along with the troubled times along the way.

I am on a stream that is turning into a river swirling around to lead me to the sea of life where I belong. An open world there for me to start exploring once again but this time with fresh eyes that open up new experiences.

When I was at university the other year studying the World of Work, I became very interested in the different types of time. *Time* became one of the topics for our writing group's homework and I decided to do a timed writing piece.

I find time a fascinating subject, a concept that is in everyone's lives. As a child I experienced it in a totally different way. A year was a very long time and the day had plenty of time for school and play. There were no time pressures as a child, our 'timetable' was worked out for us and managed by our parents. I suppose as I grew up, with the freedom to play out on the streets and downs, there must have been a time that I had to be in by, but I have no memory of such boundaries, only the boundary of where I was allowed to go. As an adult time became ruled by work and transport times. This increased tremendously as I aged, with increasing pressures in the 90's and noughties. With that came stress. But learning about time – not time management – is one of the most freeing things. To realise we have choices whether to be ruled by the clock or make time for Kairos time in our busy schedules enabling times of flow where time feels endless and there is a magical feeling of contentment and well-being.

Life exploration activity no 4

My mini storyboard (30 minutes +)

1. Take a large sheet of paper and use a landscape position.

2. Drawer four boxes across the middle of the page.

3. Choose from one of the following sets of headings and put a heading at the top of each box.
   • Spring, Summer, Autumn, Winter
   • 70's, 80's, 90's, 00's
   • Morning, Lunchtime, Afternoon, Evening
   • Yesterday, Today, Tomorrow, Next Year

4. Draw a simple picture in each box to represent a little life story inspired by the heading.

5. Share and/or write your stories.

24

FEBRUARY

FOOTPRINTS

MORNING FROST

PANCAKE PARLOUR

LIFE THROUGH THE DECADES

WHEN I DIDN'T HAVE A CLUE

ORANGE

FRIENDSHIP

MY FAVOURITE HOLIDAY DESTINATION

THE LEAP YEAR I WILL NEVER FORGET

Chapter 4

In 2017, I was researching the Sociology of Everyday Life and, in particular, belonging in relation to people, place, memories and nature. I held creative workshops as part of my dissertation project and realised I had stumbled on the key to my unique life coaching approach that had the potential to really make a difference to people's lives.

Exploring sense of belonging enables us to think about our lives from a different angle. It is something that somehow can get lost and because we may not think directly about it, we don't realise what is actually missing in our lives or what action we can take to regain or deepen our sense of belonging.

After I was made redundant, although I still kept up friendships with former colleagues, I didn't belong anymore to that work community and something was missing. I spent many a day wandering out and about. There was a local café where I felt particularly at ease. The staff were welcoming, friendly, sometimes would chat but not too intrusive. I had a warm feeling when I entered, it was like a soft blanket. I felt comfortable just sitting writing or reading a book. I would return there many times when I felt the need for that feeling. To feel I belonged.

So, within my workshops and courses, I use creative activities and topics that enable people to explore their sense of belonging. One of the first topics I may set for homework is for participants to write about nature in their lives. This can go in all sorts of directions, often taking people back to their childhood. Heather reflected on playing with a childhood friend *"Though strictly not allowed beyond these two fields, we sometimes went down the road, about a quarter of a mile away to the River Roding to catch minnows and paddle on hot summer days."* and reflecting that the man who was to become her husband in ten years' time *"could easily have been paddling and fishing downstream along the Roding Valley"*.

For myself, I gain a strong sense of belonging in relation to the sea, hearing the waves splash against the shore, the seagulls cry, the flickering light on the water, the sheer expanse of silky blue or the rough dappled crash of stormy times. I love walking on my own by the sea and letting my thoughts drift. I feel at home with the salty breeze sifting through my hair. Here is a piece of timed writing I did on *Drawn by the Sea*, the title of a book I was creating at the time with Scottish artist Stewart Morrison.

How I love the sea. Just being there. I can just stop my car by Stone Bay and I feel I am just drinking in the seascape. No matter what the weather, I just love to get out and walk. I love seeing the sea from afar and I love dipping my toes in it, rolling up my jeans and paddling in the cool sand-pillowed water.

I've gone back to Brighton now, back to my first outing on my own with a friend. I was 13 years old. We ended up on

Brighton pier. It's a special place for me. Home by the sea. Before I had my last treatment for leukaemia I went with my daughter and stayed at a hotel in a room with a sea view. It was heaven. To walk in the room and sea (sic) the bay window overlooking Brighton seafront. The traffic was rumbling past, Brighton is always busy, it's part of who it is. It's part of me. Perhaps that's why I also love going to London – the busyness, the people and the river.

Sea, river, lake, they're all special to me.

The visit to the town where I was born and grew up was very special and important to me. There was something about having my last treatment, whether I was going to survive, and I needed to go back to the place I felt I belonged. It wasn't a sad visit, we had lots of fun and met up with family so this brings back happy memories, as does the time with my friend on the pier when we went on the ghost train and my first experience of going out into the big wide world – Brighton town - without my parents.

Being in nature where there are trees and woods is also important to me. I used to walk through a park and churchyard on my way to work. I often enjoyed just looking up at the massive expanse of branches with light shimmering through the leaves on a sunny day, or carefully stepping across the fallen glowing hue of autumn, the beautiful array of colours that nature bestows on the seasonal cycle of leaves.

Extract *A day in the life* homework September 2019

Sunshine or rain, it's all part of nature and the changes in the season are what makes this country special. Everything is peaceful and there is a freshness to the day, a new start, new experiences, anticipation of the new leaf in the book.

When I asked the group to bring in an object to do with their life (or a photo of it) and write about it, Heather brought in a mouse woven out of plaited reeds. For her *"This fascinating mouse, woven out of fenland reeds, makes me think of the many strands of the last 60 plus years, woven with fun and fond memories"*. She ends up telling a story about her teenage school chums and how they still meet up yearly and *"still laugh uproariously at the day we had to rapidly exit Tate Modern when we subsided into hysterical laughter at an exhibit showing a video of a naked man, swinging his bits in time to the music"*.

My own journey back to a friendship happened when I gave the topic of Material for homework, little realising where it would take me.

Material **April 2019**

When I first suggested writing about Material for homework, in my own mind, for my own piece of writing, I was thinking I would probably write about some memento from the past that I had kept as a memory. Things that came to mind yesterday as the homework crossed my mind in passing were the jumpers that my dear mum had knitted me, proudly embellished with the 'Handmade by' labels I had given her. Then I thought, perhaps the little lilac handkerchief pouch that my mum had made for me to go in my lilac bedroom, the same material that was gathered under the handmade curtains that drew around my kidney shaped dressing table, the same material that was displayed beneath the smooth clear glass surrounded by a trim that covered the curtain-type railing. I loved that dressing table, which reminded me of my childhood bedroom, the one I had to stay in when I had childhood illnesses, particularly when I had pneumonia at five years old. My bedroom was a comfort to me but I always wanted the glass door left ajar, not shut. My window looked out onto the pond in the huge garden my parents had worked hard on to landscape. It wasn't easy for me to see the horse field and windmill opposite, which I loved and which still comes to mind when I think of home.

But, that wasn't what I decided to write about today. The material I decided to write about was the fine brown corduroy, printed with little red rosebuds and leaves. The first piece of material I bought when I started at adult education classes on dressmaking in my twenties. At the time I was commuting to London and working at BP but I still made time to go out in the evening to learn something new, this time it was dressmaking. Then, adult education was so much cheaper than it is today.

My mother-in-law did a lot of dressmaking and I always admired all the clothes she made for herself. I loved looking at dressmaking material, with all the different colours and textures. So this was my opportunity to make something. I chose to make a pinafore dress, gathered at the top of the front and back. It took me a long time to make but I persevered. Sadly, when I put it on, I didn't like it, it just didn't suit me. Or perhaps it was the corduroy that made it look as if I was nine months pregnant. It was never worn. I kept it for a while, but it was eventually disposed of.

You may think that this was a wasted class and wasted money, but on the first evening I met a new friend and we discovered that we travelled on the same train each morning. We sort of recognised each other but most people just got on the train each morning and sat quietly on their own.

From that time we started travelling together and became good friends, mainly being train buddies, until she became pregnant a couple of years later. We did keep in touch for quite a while and it was a lovely friendship, but it is one that has drifted with time. Some friendships last a lifetime, others are still special but time-limited. Each one remains as a memory that may one day be triggered by a word such as 'Material'. My needlework friend.

Life exploration activity no 5

My map of belonging

Option 1 Short version (20 minutes)

1. Take a sheet of blank A4 paper and some pens/pencils/coloured felt tips.
2. Draw a map of the places that are important to you.
3. When you have finished, straightaway set a timer for five minutes and *just write*.

Option 2 Long version (one hour +)

1. Make five separate lists:
   a. People that are, or have been, important to you.
   b. Places that are special to you, it could be countries, towns, villages, mountains, rivers, bays, beaches, buildings, homes or anywhere else.
   c. Aspects of nature that mean much to you, including pets, wildlife, flowers, trees.
   d. Significant memories that have special meaning to you.
   e. Activities that bring you a sense of belonging.
2. Using paper, pens, pencils, coloured felt tips, paints or whatever you like, create a picture map that is inspired by your lists.

Chapter 5

Receiving a personal handwritten letter is something quite special. During the first UK lockdown in 2020, Sue received a letter from a local schoolchild that moved her immensely. When replying, Sue sent one of her own fictional stories.

You may choose to write to anyone, providing an interesting perspective from which to write. You don't have to post it. You can even choose to write to yourself, whether in the present, to your younger self or your future self. Your letters can be about anything. You may wish to use it as a way to express gratitude, something which attracts increased positivity into our lives. The choice is yours.

One day the homework I set was *Write a letter to someone from your life*. One of our group wrote a letter that she decided to seal in an envelope and place in her very special journal of memories that she was passing on to her grandchildren, along with some of her other writing carried out as a result of this group.

Two of us decided to write letters to our grandmothers, Granny and Nanny. As I write this, somehow a personal letter feels very private, especially to someone who is no longer with us, even though the content may not contain any secrets. It is for this reason that I have decided not to share any extracts here, as is the choice of anyone participating in one of my workshops. Sharing is always optional

34

APRIL

NEW BEGINNINGS

SPRING

EASTER ADVENTURES

LOST IN TIME

THE MYSTERY TRAIL

FRIDAY NIGHTS

THE EGG

BLACK

SUNDAY MORNINGS

Chapter 6

Unusual questions are a sure way to send people in different directions … or so I thought! Our group seems to attract the workings of the universe, right from the very start when coincidentally all four women who joined my group had experienced the loss of their husbands within the previous year. There are other ways in which these strange occurrences happened.

One day I took in a book to show, an old one I had acquired from a second-hand book shop with an inscription inside. When Heather opened it, she experienced a strange moment seeing her mother's name handwritten inside. Although realising it had never been her own mother's book, the fact that it was the same name was an unusual experience.

Another week I passed round an art book that contained many different pictures. I asked everyone to secretly choose one picture on which to write. When it came to my turn, I opened it randomly at a picture of Honfleur in France, a place that I had wanted to visit as I knew someone who visited there often and it was where they had recently written their own book. When it came to sharing, imagine our surprise when four out of the five of us had all written about Honfleur and the only person that hadn't had thought about it.

More recently, we did some writing on *If I could acquire any one thing during 2020 that I didn't already have, what would it be* or *If I could do something different in 2020 to what I have ever done before what would it be.* Two of our members both wrote about having a caravan, not knowing previously what each other had written about.

Then there was my own piece of writing on *Somewhere I've never been to.* It really didn't occur to me that someone else would write about the moon too, but they did.

Somewhere I've never been May 2019

I've never been to the moon.

I've never been and the moon is 'somewhere'. I don't always know where it is and then it pops up in its magical way. It always intrigues me how it moves around when I am travelling yet it follows me, stalking me ahead of time …

I recall the time the other year when there was to be a special red moon, and my daughter and I were set on seeing it – at 3am in the morning! I set my alarm and got up but failed to wake my daughter from her heavy slumber. So, out into the garden I went and eventually saw it in the distance. I took a photo, I had to prove that I had seen it. It was but a small reddish dot in the night.

The first time I saw a supermoon I didn't even know it until after the event, I thought it was just in our wishful imagination.

I was sitting in my then boyfriend's car in a carpark drinking a McDonald's. It was a very special time sitting there staring up at this amazingly glowing, massive moon. We did feel that we were experiencing something unique, but it was not until the next time my boyfriend visited that he showed me the print-out he had downloaded from the internet on that supermoon …

I've never been to the moon but in my mind perhaps I have. But now I realise I haven't even written about how I came to think of the moon for my writing. The other day I paid an unexpected but hoped for visit to the Turner Contemporary and saw a unique exhibition. There were two things that really struck me – the first was a large rotating globe which reflected lights as it moved, like a disco light. On closer inspection I discovered that the globe consisted of what must have been hundreds of images of eclipses of the moon and sun. It was these that were reflected on the walls. It made the space have a tranquil quality to it. Then there was a piano playing. When I read about the music it was playing, it turned out that the music had been sent to the moon by morse code and then sent back. What was sent back had some notes missing and it was this incomplete music sent from the moon that was playing automatically on the grand piano, the notes eerily playing on their own.

38

MAY

RIPPLES OF BEAUTY

BIRTHDAYS

WHAT I HAVE LEARNT IN LIFE

THE BOOTS

SUNRISE

THE UNEXPECTED

MY CAR

SUNSHINE & SAPPHIRES

RUBY

Chapter 7

It was interesting to see the reaction of the group to the simple question *Who am I?* It may be a simple question, but I think the reality of trying to answer it is complex and also links with our sense of belonging, discussed in *Chapter 4*.

The group's perplexed response shows that our lives are in no way simple for so many reasons. I think for people of my own age and above, it is even more difficult. We have seen so much change in our one life, in the world, society and the way in which it impacts on our lives. In this chapter I share the response of one member of our group.

Who am I? Sue pre-March 2020

I'm a 74 year old widow, mother and grandmother. OMG is that who I really am. Sounds boring doesn't it?

I don't think I'm boring although I do go on a bit. I'd like to think I was eccentric but have never quite had the nerve to carry it off.

I think I'm kind and considerate up to a point but I don't seem to have as much patience with others as I used to when I was young.

When I was young I was still me. Do we change when we get older?

I've always been sensitive and still am. I've become more creative but then I have more time now.

Back to the question 'who' am I? Not what or why but who.

If the question was what am I that would be easier 'I'm a human being – female' and why - that's difficult why are we? There must be a reason why we are here. I've not yet figured out that reason.

Back to who:-

I'm not just a female person, I'm a very complicated mixture made up of thoughts, experiences, luck, fate, relationships, encounters - life.

The sliding door - if my Mum and Dad hadn't moved to Herne Bay I'd never have met Barry and moved to Acol, had children, gone to work, travelled abroad, had grandchildren and become who I am today.

A 74 year old widow, mother and grandmother.

Written on Minnis Bay seafront on Sunday with the wind blowing and waves crashing onto the sand.

When I was bringing the draft of this book together, I asked Sue if she would be happy to write a reflection on the foregoing. This is what she wrote.

Sue's reflections a few months later

Several months after I wrote the above we find ourselves, unbelievably, in the midst of a global pandemic – Coronavirus.

I'm back at my favourite beachside location, again it's windy and the waves crashing on the shore.

It's quiet today a few cyclists and windsurfers and one or two families on the beach social distancing of course.

The tide comes in and goes out as it has done for centuries and will continue to do so whatever happens to us.

I'm another year older, 75 now. Still the same person but more anxious and worried about the future. I've lost a few friends lately, some too early some expected. It's inevitable when we reach my age.

I'm 'at risk' and had a letter from the Government telling me this. I didn't need a letter. I know I have health issues. Another reason to be anxious.

We are all going to die sometime, that's a certainty, but when and how – that's the worry.

Who am I today?

Still me – a 75 year old widow, mother and grandmother!

42

JUNE

STRAWBERRY JAM

GRASS

ANIMALS

MY SPECIAL TALENTS

WHEN I WENT CAMPING

THE BROKEN DOOR

EMERALD

THE TOP OF THE TREE

MOON

Chapter 8

Sometimes writing about life can become blurred with fiction, as in a dream. Other times we can deliberately set out to mix things up a bit and write life story fiction.

The Circus Sue

As soon as I was old enough to leave school I left home and joined a circus.

I wanted to travel and have some fun and excitement so I was full of enthusiasm until they made me share a caravan with a fortune teller whose crystal ball predicted my career would end in tears.

However I turned up for work on Day 1 and was given a shovel and bucket and was told to muck out the horses.

I like animals at a distance but horses can be unpredictable and rather large and cleaning up round them a dangerous occupation. One day I left the stable door open and one got out so I was swiftly demoted to picking up litter from the grounds after the show had finished.

Neither of these jobs were exactly what I had in mind.

I rather imagined I would be given a starring role in the ring with a uniform, short skirt, fishnet tights. I would have been happy even to sit in the box office handling cash and issuing tickets.

I mentioned this to the ring master one day who laughed in my face. Just who do you think you are, you've only been here 5 minutes.   It takes years of experience before I let you near members of the public'.

Maybe I'd made a bad decision after all, what should I do?

The French Foreign Legion hadn't been on my list given to the Careers Officer at School.   It had been Hairdresser, Nurse or Secretary so I left the circus and went to college.

Many secretarial jobs followed over the next 40 years, working for Accountant, Builders Merchant, Foundry, Estate Agent, Solicitor, Hospital and more.

Maybe if I'd persevered you could have seen me riding bareback or swinging from a trapeze in a skimpy costume.

Who knows?

Life exploration activity no 6

My dream journey

Think of a dream journey (no limitations, forget about time and cost and any other restricting factors). My map of belonging (p31) coupled with online research and browsing through magazines will help with inspiration.

Option 1 Vision boarding (two hours +)

1. Take time to gather images that you love related to your dream journey. Include those that express feelings and activities along the way, people, places, transport, culture, the senses, nature. You may choose to create some of your own images or use your own photos.
2. Create your vision board. It is important to find a time when you can relax without any pressures so that you gain maximum benefit using a mindful approach, without any distractions. You can either cut and paste, draw or paint onto a large sheet of paper or card, or use computer software to produce a digital picture.

Option 2 Letter inviting your future companion (one hour +)

1. Give yourself a different name and decide who, or what, will be your companion.
2. Write a long letter inviting your companion telling them in detail about your future journey plans and what you hope to do. Let them know why you would like to invite them and what you think they would enjoy about joining you for the journey. Tell them why this dream journey means so much to you.

46

JULY

THE BEACH HUT

THE MIRROR

A BRIEF ENCOUNTER

SKIPPING

MIDNIGHT

WHITE

NOTE TO A FRIEND

WHEN I DID SOMETHING UNEXPECTED

THE BEAUTY OF THE DAY

Chapter 9

I set *The Enchanted Garden* for homework when we were due to meet at a wonderful hotel by Botany Bay the following week. It seemed to lead each of us to quite a special place. Here are two pieces I wrote myself, the second piece is a reflection on the first.

The Enchanted Garden July 2019

(1)

The waves lap against the shore. I'm lying on the soft sun lounger, the sun providing a warm cloak. My eyes are closed as I listen to the distant sound of summer. Birds chirping, seagulls swimming through the air. I drift off into a lazy slumber.

Awakening, I become aware of a new sensation. I can feel silent tickles on my skin. Slowly opening my eyes I catch sight of purple petals flowing over me. High above the lofty branches of trees are staring down at me. I look, not comprehending what I am seeing. Am I still asleep? Am I dreaming? I turn to the ground beside me and the golden shafts of sand remain.

Yet there it is before me. Memories of a much-loved garden as real today as it was then. The hard work must have taken many years. Each level was landscaped. Each one had a rockery, lawn, walls and crazy paving. Then there was the pond with the weeping willow draping over it that I could see from my bedroom window. The garden swept down the side of the bungalow and was a beautiful sight with so many flowers, particularly roses and the little 'bunny' flowers.

As I sit, the tide comes in, sweeping over the crazy paving, refreshing the memories of so long ago. The waves wash over the flowers and leaves and the water lilies bobble on the surface.

My enchanted garden lives with the sea, encompassing all that I love. Magical. Surreal. Forever mine to treasure.

(2)

The Enchanted Garden means many things to me. It sounds like a fairy story and that takes me back to my childhood. It takes me home to where I belonged. Whilst my bedroom was my special space, with my toys, the kidney-shaped and lilac-draped dressing table and the glass door that used to be left ajar while I listened to the radio before I slept, it is the garden that stands out beyond all.

The bungalow was surrounded by large gardens on three sides, back, side and front. The back garden was our private family garden, the one where I tried to learn to ride an old red bicycle and failed, never to ride again until I rode a motorbike aged 18. The side garden swept down the hill, layered and manicured with large mountainous rocks, colourful flowers, curvy-shaped pond, weeping willow and crazy paving paths and matching little walls. The front garden merged with it and presented a display of hydrangeas and the garage with drive.

What made it so special is that it was created with love and toil by my parents and the foundations of their crazy paved design remains today (at least till about five years ago when I last saw it). Whilst mum and dad lovingly created the garden in their last home, it did not offer the opportunity to shape it in the way they did at Mill Rise with the mounds of earth being shifted creating mountains to climb in my memory mind.

Somehow, when I think of my own homes I have lived in, it is the garden I remember the best. Perhaps it is the connection with nature that it enables and why I always hope to have a garden of some kind. Perhaps it is the memories of playing with a puppy in our first home, our children splashing around having fun in a paddling pool, mum coming round with boxes of beautiful plants and transforming our front garden, summer family gatherings with the trailer tent opened up.

Even when I stayed in hospital when I was ill, it was to the special garden I would go to escape if I could and look up to the clouds, enjoy the plants tended by volunteers and sit listening to the sounds of nature.

I recall one home I lived in for a few years felt magical. There were no special plants or special layout, it was turfed with shrubs that looked after themselves. But it was the massive trees that spread across the wide width of the garden, the squirrels, bird song and the feeling that I was in the middle of the countryside yet in fact living at the end of a close in a built-up area ...

Once again I live in a house whose garden gives me that countryside feel, and now I have a title for a special painting I have. Encouraged by my artist friend, I set myself up to paint en plein air to capture the essence of this garden, I enjoyed mixing the colours and spreading them with thought and care over the canvas as I connected with nature ...

So, what the Enchanted Garden means to me is something, a feeling, that encompasses my mum's deep love of gardening, a feeling of home and my love of nature. It is a feeling of belonging and a sense of peace and whenever I visit a garden when I am out and about, this feeling is recreated and will never leave me.

Another member of the group wrote a very personal and moving piece of her own on The Enchanted Garden, one that seemed to symbolise her experiences and feelings about the loss of her husband and yet how he still remained with her, now and into the future as she lived her own life. It felt somewhat comforting as an observer privileged to share in such a heartfelt piece of writing. Here is an extract from the longer piece.

The Enchanted Garden Heather

Finally light shone at the end of the tunnel and just ahead of her she saw him seated on a beautiful, ornate bench, silhouetted against the sparkling, singing streams of water cascading down a rock of diamond, white marble.

It was such a relief to see him there, to know he was safe. The panic she had known, the emptiness, the fear of never finding him again was gone. She walked slowly toward him.

'At last! Where have you been' he said gently in his so familiar, calm voice. 'I've been worried about you'.

'Oh I've been a bit lost, I think. I've been looking for you and trying to imagine where you had got to' she said.

He smiled, 'I'm here most days, it's so calm and peaceful and safe.'

'Can't I stay here in this lovely garden too? I don't have to get back. I worry about leaving you here.'

'You don't need to worry about me. When you close your eyes you will always feel the warmth, smell the scent and see me here. You will feel my love around you. I'll be waiting for you, there's no need to rush. You've got lots to do yet and you can join me when you're ready.' He gave that lovely, calm and gentle half smile as he turned to watch the birds fly off toward the trees.

She felt the sun on her face and smelt a strong scent as she opened her eyes. She wasn't panicked, she was calm as she got out of bed, looked out of the window and remembered where she was, Westgate on Sea. Heath Park Road was 4 years and 180 miles away. The sparkling sea and the infinite horizon stretched before her. She had lots to do.

AUGUST

THE FIELD OF FUN

THE CAMPERVAN

THE SEA SHELL

SUNSET

WHEN I SLEPT UNDER THE STARS

THE MOUNTAIN OF MY DREAMS

BANK HOLIDAY BLUNDERS

BLUE

MY CRAZY ADVENTURE

Chapter 10

The Magic Carpet was one of the last themes set for homework in March 2020 before lockdown and Sue enjoyed sharing her story.

The Magic Carpet Sue March 2020 (pre-lockdown)

I do actually have a magic carpet, I keep it in the shed. I don't normally tell people about it as they may want to borrow it.

Last time I lent it to somebody they took it – or it took them – to Switzerland where it got stuck in a snowdrift and it was weeks before I got it back.

After Barry died, I went to the Maldives on it – he would never go there as he said we would get bored. He was right – I did get bored – a month later!

I often use it to go to Tesco. It's handy for shopping and there's a special place for them round the back.

I go to London too – it doesn't take long and it's easier than being stuck in traffic.

Last time I landed on the roof of Buckingham Palace and watched the Changing of the Guard. I've been to Putney Bridge to watch the Boat Race and another time stopped in the grounds of the Chelsea Hospital for the Chelsea Flower Show.

The possibilities for its use are endless. It can go back or forward in time. I'm a bit nervous about doing that as I might get stuck in the 60's or something. I wouldn't want to have been 75 in 1964 it was much more fun being 19!

I've never done anything illegal on it but considered that if I ever became short of money I could always go into the vaults of the Bank of England and help myself. If I get caught and put in Prison, I could easily fly out again.

After I die, I'd like to leave it to the Red Cross who could use it to send supplies to War Torn Countries, or airlift children to safety.

Meanwhile I'm just continuing using it whenever I'm at a loose end.

Today I've got to leave early as I'm going to a retirement party.

Sorry – I must fly!!!

For myself, this writing prompt took me on a journey through my memories to a special home.

The magic carpet swings forward and back as its tufts play with the hopes and memories in my mind. When I first think of a Magic Carpet I think of it taking me wherever I might wish to go, flying high in the sky, soaring across the hilly mounds below as it sweeps up into the air amidst the birds and clouds on a bright summer's day, the wavy shoreline etched alongside the turquoise pool of sea glistening in the air.

Yet it also takes me back to a time in my life when I lived in one of the first homes of my own that I loved. The carpet that brought our dreams of a beautiful lounge complete. The one that also had a turquoise hue sprinkled with gold and adorned with floral designs. The one that my feet melted into, that stood the test of time over the years when our children grew up from babes gurgling as they lay on their backs, smiling and playing to school children romping around. The Christmas tree presents piled on top while they lay sleeping above in their beds, their stockings awaiting them. This was a carpet reminiscent of a family tradition, a quality Axminster set to last a lifetime and now a lifetime of memories.

As it rises up into the sky it takes with it the beautiful home I lived in for about seventeen years, the longest by far in any one place – ever.

SEPTEMBER

DAWN

A MEMORABLE BREAK

THE CAFE THAT NEVER CLOSED

PINK

A SPECIAL MEMORY

WHEN I JUST HAD TO SAY "YES!"

THE TREE HOUSE

AUTUMN

THE ROAD TRIP

Chapter 11

As a topic *Things that lighten my mood and people that bring me joy* gets people thinking about what makes them feel good. It helps raise self-awareness and perhaps to realise that they don't allow enough time for things that they really enjoy doing and seeing people that are important to them and for their own well-being.

Here is my own piece of homework which I wrote when visiting one of my favourite hotels just to sit with a hot chocolate, reflect on life and write. I always try to have a pen and notepad with me for whenever I feel the urge to write something down.

Things that lighten my mood

Walking along by the seaside with not a care in the world. No matter what else is going on, when I find myself alongside the sea my mood lifts. Be it rain or shine, the effect is the same though the best is ambling along with the sun glistening down on the sea and a gentle breeze brushing past me, washing away my cares.

At home it is a family album filled with snapshots from happy times, whether it be memories of childhood or my children being born and growing up. Holiday times across the years. It reinforces what is important.

Getting up from a seat and striding towards the dance floor, immersing myself in the music and getting lost in the rhythm and atmosphere of the moment. Taking a seat and the curtains opening on a live music concert. Just thoughts of these times in the past can lift my mood.

Then it comes to living in the now, right here, this moment. Focussing on breathing in and out with my eyes closed, releasing any tension in my body. Becoming aware of my surroundings, letting all the things I have been thinking or worrying about drift from my mind. Allowing myself to be lost in peace.

Lighting a candle and sitting watching it flicker in the soft lighting that it spreads across the room. Picking up a brush, squeezing out colours onto a palette, mixing them with a dab of water and seeing the magic that happens as different shades emerge. Spreading the colours across the paper, allowing my creativity to run wild.

Lifting the lid on a piano, tentatively trying out a few notes, trying to play from music and enjoying the moment there on my own. Exploring a new path, a new place, allowing my feet the freedom to walk wherever they please, the discoveries that are made, the sights, the sounds, the smells. Getting on a train, taking my seat and gently stirring with the rhythm of the rails, reaching a familiar or new destination.

Planning a holiday, an adventure, for some future time whenever that may be with intrigue, excitement, hope and dreams. Exploring opportunities for new learning, new experiences that open up new worlds to me. These are just some of the things that lighten my mood.

People that bring me Joy

I had to stop and think for a moment about the meaning of joy. After googling several meanings my own definition is an internal feeling of great happiness, in this case caused by certain people. Mostly I think of my children, the intensity of feelings of happiness. Yet this also extends to personal relationships when they have been at their highest level of compatibility and love. There have been certain moments in life when I have experienced sheer joy in the moment as a result of the people around me. This has included the birth of my children, getting married and experiencing others close to me getting married. Included within these moments are times when I have had such a wonderful time with someone that I am in love with, that special closeness and intimacy, that can just be a touch, a look. Fleeting moments of joy have been experienced on the dance floor, walking home hand in hand after a great night out or having a good laugh with friends.

So, the people that bring me joy are those that I feel a special closeness with, experiencing fun, laughter, friendship and love. The sharing of experiences where all else is put aside and those that truly matter are given the time they deserve. Joy is not something that can be planned for, but it happens when we discover what truly brings us happiness and share those moments with friends and family that make us feel special.

Joy comes from the special memories of those moments with people who matter to us, now or in the past, for whatever reason. The feelings of joy can linger on and be rekindled whether we are still with that person or not.

I even begin to feel joyful just by thinking about joy. Life is full of riches that have nothing to do with money and materialism. We all have the capacity for joy if we can just find the key to unlock that special place of feeling.

OCTOBER

THE WITCH

THE RING

THE DANCING TREE

HALLOWEEN TALES

DUSK

WAVES OF WONDER

A BIG HUG WAS ALL I NEEDED

GREEN

A PEACEFUL RETREAT

Chapter 12

The benefits of using a positive life story coaching approach to empower people to communicate with both themselves and others, and to share their stories, enables time for everyone to learn from and inspire each other with their ideas.

Alongside the recognition of common experiences, there is also a shared understanding that each person's experience is different. Everyone is on their own journey at their own pace, taking the next step when they are ready.

During the time that our group were meeting, Sue started having holidays on her own, something that she had previously found it difficult to consider, and now enjoys planning her future holidays.

Sue

I joined Kay's course because I wanted to write a journal about my life and needed a bit of motivation. There are just four of us on the course. We are all women, retired and all recently widowed. At our first meeting, Kay introduced herself and we were soon put at ease. She explained that the course would encourage writing and with the aid of the 'Life Wheels' etc certain areas of our lives which maybe we were less than happy with could be improved and also highlighting people, places and things which are important to us improving our general well-being.

As the course progressed (four months longer than the original eight weeks) Kay suggested topics to write about. She is a very good listener and we talked a lot about our life now, our families and our husbands. We laughed, we cried and our friendship grew.

The course wasn't planned as a bereavement group but as we had all been touched by death it soon became apparent that it was what we all needed.

Kay's experiences and training plus sensitivity make her the ideal person to give advice and guidance and dealing with bereavement and other sensitive issues.

On a personal note, I'm slowly coming to terms with the fact that becoming widowed has two sides to it.

1) *Losing a husband, missing him and feeling sad that he's gone*

BUT

2) *Life goes on. My life has changed. I have friends and family but they have their own lives. Yes I spend time with them but I am now on my own.*

I've started doing more on my own, days out and even holidays, and I enjoy it.

SN August 2019

Life exploration activity no 7

My life wheel (30 minutes +)

This coaching tool has the most impact when carried out face to face, either in one of my workshops or one to one. I hope the following will enable you to try it out for yourself and is a reminder for those who have joined me online or in person.)

1. Think about what makes up your life. List up to eight areas, eg health, work, family, friends, home, leisure, hobbies, wealth, creativity. It is important to come up with your own list, your life is unique.

2. On a large sheet of paper, at the top write the heading "My life wheel (and today's date)". Draw a large circle, divide it into eight segments (like cutting a cake). Around the outside of the circle, head up each segment with the items in your list.

3. Ask yourself "How satisfied am I with this area of my life?" Score each segment separately on a scale 1 to 10, 1 = not satisfied at all, 10 = perfect.

4. Pick three segments you would like to focus on ... then pick just one of the three. (You can repeat the exercise with the other segments, but action taken in one area of your life can have a beneficial impact on the others.)

5. With your one chosen segment, imagine and dream with NO LIMITS what that area of your life would be like if it was a perfect 10. Then, *just write* (or draw) for a minimum of five minutes.

6. Choose one small action that you could take now or this week to move you towards the perfect 10.

64

NOVEMBER

THE PYJAMA PARTY

MUDDY ADVENTURES

THE MANTELPIECE

MY FAVOURITE BLANKET

CHOCOLATE

FIREWORKS

WHAT FAMILY MEANS TO ME

RED

AN UNEXPECTED GUEST

Chapter 13

I trained as a life coach over fifteen years ago. The training changed my life and the way I approached things. It also resulted in my being successful in getting a totally different job that I loved working for a local charity which I did for the next eight years.

Now, as a Life Story Empowerment Coach, I believe in enabling people to tell their stories in a way that acknowledges their past yet empowers them to live their life in a way that will bring them a sense of fulfilment and joy.

My years of listening to people in different capacities, especially as a mediator in the community and working with young people and their families, have shown me that the stories behind people's lives are so different to the problems that they bring on the surface, and in some cases heart-rending, more than anyone could imagine. I have learnt not to make assumptions about people. We never know what they are going through, the life they have led.

There are always life challenges that keep coming our way, but it is how we choose to deal with things that is important and to recognise that sometimes difficult times can end up enriching our lives. We see what wonderful people we have around us who are happy to listen and really care about us. We value the special moments, the little things.

The way in which I run my writing groups, workshops and courses specifically excludes any critiquing by either myself or other participants. That has been a personal choice I have made based on the kind of experience I wish to offer. I am qualified to teach but I am not a creative writing teacher and am certainly not an expert. My experience of mediation has opened my eyes to the benefits of allowing people to feel safe and to not feel judged. This enables people to enjoy sharing their writing and be listened to, without having to worry about whether the way in which they have written it is right or wrong. It is *their* story to be told as *they wish* to tell it.

I fully recognise that critiquing has a valuable part to play in the right learning environment and for a specific purpose. I myself attended a wonderful creative writing course with an inspirational teacher as part of an Access to University course after I was made redundant from the job that I loved. Not only did this reveal to me the benefits of creativity and writing, together with coming together as a special group, it was also my route to being a very mature student studying for a Bachelor of Science degree in Social Sciences. This degree was about life, it was so diverse and interesting and covered so many things I was interested in. My dissertation was on sense of belonging, and I carried out qualitative research involving creative workshops – writing and drawing. This highlighted for me the importance of people, place, memories and nature. Combined with my coaching skills and previous work experience, this new learning has led to my personal approach of Life Story Writing.

I have a real passion for what I do, and an important part of that is bringing people together and enabling a relaxed and social time in which to share. By facilitating workshops and courses, people are empowered to come together and learn from each other, making new connections and friendships along the way.

The aim of this book was to celebrate the creation of our wonderful writing group, and at the same time to inspire others to write and share the little stories about their lives.

The stories we tell about our life, whether to ourselves or to others, enable us to acknowledge our feelings and what has happened to us, to explore what is really important and enable us to consider what might be helpful. Are we focussing too much on the negative and not allowing all the good things that have happened to us to be given credit?

Expressing gratitude every day for the good things in our lives in itself can prove life-changing, bringing positive things into our lives rather than attracting negativity. The use of the life wheel coaching tool can help us create stories about our future lives, to dream without limits and live life to the full.

By telling our stories, we start to realise what truly matters to us. By visualising the ideal life and telling an inspirational story about our future, it can lift our spirits, help motivate us and lend direction for the little steps along the way.

Life doesn't have to be perfect. It is in the imperfections that we find new learning and insight. Despite the troubles of the pandemic, nothing can take away the memories of experiences that have brought joy to our hearts together.

Life exploration activity no 8

My pot of gratitude and joy (30 minutes + ongoing)

1. Choose a special pot (or box) with a lid that you could use to place bits of paper in. This can be clear glass or decorative and big enough for you to put your hand in it. (Alternatively use a special box which can be one that you decorate yourself.)

2. Cut up squares of paper large enough to write three lines or a sentence or two on (ideally use two different colour papers – one for gratitude and one for joy but this is not essential).

3. Every morning and/or evening use a separate piece of paper to write on for the following and add them to the pot or box:
   a. Three things that I am grateful for
   b. Something that brings me joy

4. If you find yourself stuck, take five minutes just to relax and breathe then look around you for the tiniest things, indoors or outdoors, that you are grateful for or that bring you joy.

5. On the days when you are stuck for what to pop in the pot, enjoy randomly picking two pieces of paper (one of each colour if you have them) and spend a few moments reflecting on their content. Also consider reading Chapter 11 (page 57) and looking back on Life exploration activities numbers 2, 3 and 5 (see pages 9, 15 and 31).

70

DECEMBER

THE GLOWING LIGHT

I REMEMBER WHEN I SANG CAROLS

WINTER

BAUBLES GALORE

A POEM

THE CHRISTMAS PARTY

THE ROBIN

PUDDINGS & PIES

A LETTER TO THE POST-PERSON

Chapter 14

My Life Story Writing method is illustrated by the Waves and Pebbles Kite that will be explored in a future publication along with the way in which I use the life wheel coaching tool to inspire writing about our dreams for the future. It offers something different that is for anyone regardless of whether or not they wish to be a writer. Despite the name, there is no requirement to actually *write* – drawing, symbols or any other creative method is equally effective as it is the meaning to yourself and the sharing with others that is most important.

Life Story Writing is a way to enjoy recalling and sharing the little stories in life with the opportunity to experience an increased sense of well-being through the connections being made. Whilst living through the pandemic has been (and still is at the time of publication) such a difficult and challenging time, and many people have sadly been affected by the loss of loved ones, or the loss of good health, jobs or businesses, I hope that you may be able to capture some of the special moments that you have experienced during this time, maybe something new you have tried, looking more closely at the nature in your garden, walks you have had, a new hobby or the different ways you have celebrated special occasions. Don't forget to enjoy writing about your dreams for the future no matter how farfetched or distant they may seem. There is much joy to be found in both writing and planning and the clearer we become about what we would like and write it down, the more likely it is to happen.

I would love to hear from you with any stories or experiences you would like to share that have been triggered by discovering our book, however short or small they may be. The little things can make the biggest difference to our lives.

As I finish writing these last words, it is with grateful thanks to four very special women, Sue, Heather, Jenny and Jeanie, who I had the greatest privilege to meet in January 2019 and have spent so many hours with. The creation of our Life Story Writing friendship group has been one of the most special experiences of my life that I will never forget. We have had such fun together, with many special moments and enjoyed sharing so many stories and you have all helped my dream to come true. I truly hope that in some way, as we are each starting out on our new journeys, and as we emerge from the disruption of the lockdowns, that our group will be reborn in some way and that we may one day create another book, perhaps *Writing Back to Happiness Revisited* or whatever title emerges when spending magic time together.

Much love to all.

Kay

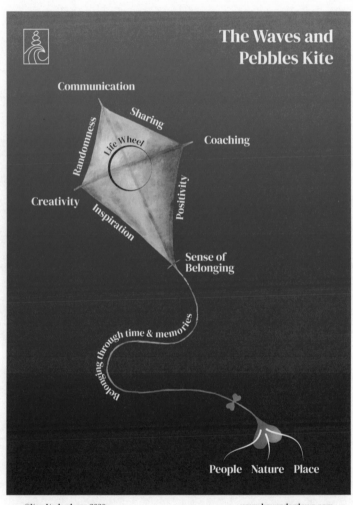

©Kay Underdown 2020

74

NEW YEAR

REFLECTIONS

PURPLE

TIME

THIS IS ME!

THE ROAD AHEAD

SPARKLE

A LETTER TO THE REAL ME

CELEBRATING LIFE

BUDDING DREAMS

Afterword - holding on, letting go

I had been waiting for the perfect way to end this book, a representation of something that has been a very special period of my life. Somehow, I found myself putting it off, holding back from the inevitable. I thought that I could bring the book to a grand finale, share the last best bits. I have found this difficult to do amongst the turmoil of life over the past 18 months, the right words just haven't come and the weekly connections which I valued so much are no longer there. I thought I had to write something perfect, and this stopped me from picking up my pen.

This reinforces a message that needs to be included within this book and of which I sometimes need to be reminded myself. Don't let any limiting thoughts stop you from going on your own Life Story Writing adventure, whether on your own, with friends or, like us, with a random group that somehow came together through a sequence of events that conspired to work their magic. Yes, it felt like magic and turned into a dream, bringing together what I believe in and enabling me to do something I really love and to share it with others who have become my friends.

So now is the time to let go. We have journeyed together, gone down many roads and explored different paths, leading to numerous surprise rabbit holes. Life is a world of stories, and the best ones start with you and your loved ones, whether here in the present, within your heartfelt memories, or in your hopes and dreams for the future.

I hope you will discover that Life Story Writing is a gift you can give to yourself however you wish to use it. In sharing your stories at a small get-together, with strangers or with friends, that is your gift to others. You are sharing your joy, love of life, humour, hobbies, curiosity and philosophy of life, along with any sadness or other emotions that ripple through our lives. The multiplicity of life touches us all in different ways and enables us to connect on such a special level.

My last request to my ladies was to write about their favourite flowers and to tell me their favourite trees. I had the book cover in mind but more importantly I feel that there was a message within this. It is about growth and beauty, the different shapes and shades of our lives, and within this most especially is about having the hope and trust to do all you can to nurture something but then to be able to let go and allow it to grow in its own beautiful way.

My favourite flower Sue

My favourite flower has to be the Rose since my maiden name was Rose – Susan Rose. I liked my name until I attended Secondary School and my Headmaster's name was also Rose. I was shy and was horrified as my classmates thought I was his daughter. ... I discovered recently through Social Media that Mr Rose's father was Bishop of Dover and further research revealed he was Bishop when I was confirmed a year before. I'm sure my parents knew this but didn't tell me. ... Family funerals feature Roses in the wreaths, we can't possibly use any other flowers!

Roses are pretty, delicate, perfumed and varied – there are climbers, ramblers, standard, bush, shrub and wild plus many more. They flower abundantly from early Summer in a choice of colours - pastel shades of pink, peach, cream or white and vibrant yellow and gold, orange, crimson and red.

(Sue lists some of the women who have had Roses named after them.)

The list is endless.

I wonder what I'd have to do to have a rose named after me? Marry a Prince, write a book, star in a film – it's probably too late for that now but at least I started life as a Rose!

My favourite flower Jenny

How do I choose my favourite flower? It seems an impossible task as each flower, as it comes into season, becomes the favourite. The excitement of seeing that first snowdrop after a long cold winter telling us that Spring is just around the corner, followed by the crocus and shortly afterwards the daffodils that are not at all put off by a late frost or even snow — how can I choose between them? I do love the tall stately tulips that always seem to bloom for a number of weeks in a wonderful range of colours. Two years ago now when we took days out for granted I visited Hever Castle with friends to see the tulips. It was a wonderful display and the day was made even more special by the walk we took through the bluebell woods nearby bringing back memories of the times when Charles used to take us out every Spring to see the bluebells in the woods near Canterbury. He always said it was for me but I know it was just as much for him as we stood and gazed at the lovely carpet of bluebells spread out under the trees in front of us.

However, a choice must be made between these flowers and all those that haven't been named and my choice has to be the rose as my number one favourite. When we see the beautiful blooms and smell the intoxicating perfume of the rose then we know that it is truly summer. Summertime with its long sunny days sitting in the garden under the shade of my cherry tree with the roses in bloom just a few feet away has to be the best time. Either alone with a good book or with family and friends enjoying tea and cake, these are days to treasure and remember in the long winter months ahead. The rose symbolises these special times to me and has to be my very favourite flower.

My favourite flower **Heather**

My favourite flower is a very simple one, the bluebell. There are many reasons for this lowly choice. Apart from its beauty, it is self sufficient and wondrously comes back cheerfully every year without any need for assistance from gardeners. At the first fledgling hints of Spring its flower spikes begin to swell and grow upwards to the light until, with a little bit of sun, it bursts out among the waking trees, frothy with green buds and blossoms, in patches of woodland across the land.

In some ways it is a symbol of renewal, it springs up, gives joy and brightens the world, but it has its season and must die, but like hope it springs eternal and is back the next year.

You cannot beat the intensity of its natural perfume. Strong and sweet and somehow refreshing and yet calming all in one hit. When I come across a carpet of bluebells and the scent hits me it brings back such happy times on long woodland walks with Alan, when we often smelled them before we even saw them. I used to take my mum and Alex, her 'man' and to me the grandad I never really had, on Spring drives to see the wonderful sight of woodlands with bright blue, tree to tree carpets. We loved the sight and smell and would celebrate on the way home with a McFlurry!!!

We reminisced about this often, especially when they were no longer able to go to see them.

As a child I holidayed in Scotland every summer. It was a chance for my mum to visit her family, but it was also wonderful for us. The freedom, the fun we had and the welcome we got was lovely. We came to consider ourselves as 'wee lassies'. I learnt to play the piano from the age of 6 or 7 and one of the first 'real' pieces I could play was ... (Scottish and the chorus includes both heather and the bluebell). *So I was regularly trotted out to play it at family gatherings.*

I can't see bluebells without thinking of those times, or smell their unique scent without bringing back those lovely moments with those who mean so much to me.

The pandemic hit and splattered our lives. We've had to bring it back together, not quite as it was before. But alongside that is a wealth of different stories and experiences to be told, your own history of an unprecedented time. You may choose to tell it or to move on.

I am so glad to say that at the time of writing, Jenny, Jeanie, Sue and Heather have now resumed their meetings at our usual hotel, together with their special homemade biscuits, and it was a touching moment for me to be able to join them online from afar and say hello.

Life goes on even when we are not there and I believe that the sharing of our stories strengthens our connection with others and the places that are important to us, building our resilience to live our own lives.

This book is my gift to my friends, their gift to me and it's our gift to you. Let us all enjoy sharing the little stories in life that bring us together.

Kay, Sue, Jenny, Heather & Jeanie

January 2022

SPRING

MY NEW PROJECT

RAINBOW

SPARKLING ROBES

WHAT I NEVER THOUGHT I'D HAVE OR DO

IF I KNEW WHAT I WANTED TO DO I WOULD ...

BLUEBELLS IN THE SAND

YELLOW

THE BOX

MY TREASURE TROVE FOR THE FUTURE

Waves and Pebbles Publishing is my own publishing imprint. Other publications include:

Life Happens Live Happy (2019). Based on Kay's own experience of being diagnosed with Acute Promyelocytic Leukaemia and aimed at anyone going through disruption in their life that is affecting their well-being. Inspiring the use of writing, creativity and a positive approach to life, appreciating the little things along the way.

Books created in collaboration with Scottish artist Stewart Morrison:

Drawn by the Sea - a collaborative art project The Isle of Thanet (2019). Inspired originally by Kay carrying out a visual sociology assignment at Stone Bay in Broadstairs and communicating with Stewart about what she could see.

Drawn by the Sea 2020 Scottish Coastal Communities. A journey around the coast of Scotland in words and pictures. A book Stewart and I decided to create together during the lockdowns of 2020 based on a journey that Stewart was aiming to do and including places he had already visited.

Forthcoming

Bella and Bobbles A children's story about a chocolate Labrador and a baby Seagull. A little story about dealing with change, friendship and loss inspired by a move to the Isle of Thanet coast.

To learn a little more about me, please do visit my Waves and Pebbles blog, Random thoughts and writing on life, memories and creativity, with a variable regularity of posts from 2015 onwards.

www.wavesandpebbles.blog

A space for me to record the little stories
I wish to share with my family and friends
(written and unwritten)

A space for me to write and draw

the little things that bring me joy